Contents

Chapter		Page
1.	My Story	4
2.	What is Chi Gung?	16
3.	An Overview of Chi Gung	28
4.	Some Chi Gung History	37
5.	Modern Teachers	44
6.	A Basic Breathing Practice	53
7.	What is Shibashi?	57
8.	Fundamentals of Shibashi	65
9.	Shibashi Teachers	70
10.	The Future	79
	Bibliography	89

Preface

Chi Gung is the ancient art of moving, breathing and focusing your mind. When you practise regularly, your mind will gradually become calm and peaceful, and your whole being will start to feel more harmonised and balanced. Through sensing and feeling, and examining your inner experiences, you will start to understand yourself physically and mentally.

You don't need to be super fit to practice Chi Gung. You don't need to wear any special clothes or uniform. Improve your level of health and well-being no matter what level you're at. *Always seek the advice of a healthcare specialist before undertaking any exercise.*

I have compiled this book from the wisdom and experiences of a select group of masters and teachers I admire. I have also acknowledged all sources of information as accurately and sincerely as I can. If you see some words of yours in this book, that I have not acknowledged, then I apologise in advance.

I have been practicing Chi Gung for 25 years and teaching for over 20 years. It has been my privilege to learn from top masters from all over the world. With my daily teaching, my intention is to honour all Chi Gung traditions whilst also moving forward with intelligence, intellect and vision.

In this book you will encounter different ways to spell Chi Gung (pronounced Chee *Gong*). Literally "Life

Energy Cultivation", a practice of aligning breath, movement, and awareness. Here is a sample of the spellings. Chi Kung, Chi *Gong*, *Qi Gong*.

Chi Gung can be a life time study. Togetherness and community can be created with group Chi Gung practice. Paradoxically and powerfully we also develop aloneness whilst we practice.

This book is designed to educate and inform you about the profound art form of Chi Gung. Also to enthuse you to take up and practice the powerful Chi Gung movements called 'Shibashi Exercises'.

Remember, when you practice the Shibashi exercises, to make things simple for yourself, and most importantly, enjoy what you are doing. In any art or discipline, progress and achievement come naturally through perseverance.

I'd like to thank Chi Gung students all over the world. Your dedication and practice not only greatly benefits your health and wellbeing, but contributes to the continual development of this beautiful and powerful art.

Michael Richards
Chi Gung and Tai Chi Teacher
BA (hons) Leisure Management

Chapter 1

My Story

"What you practise you surely become" – San Gee Tam, Founder of the Golden Flower Tai Chi Association

In the past I've been a bit of a 'purist' whilst learning and teaching Chi Gung, Tai Chi and 'Internal Alchemy'. By 'purist' I mean teaching a small number of people the incredibly long, personal and sometimes arduous process of learning how to transform their health and well-being, using the principles and practice of Chi Gung and Tai Chi.

For many years I diligently practiced my Tai Chi, learning from experts and Tai Chi Masters. My progress was gradual. Step by step I successfully transformed my body, which was a fit and healthy one, into a body that was also a relaxed and powerful one.

My first teacher Sangeetam (James Holland) always included Chi Gung with his Tai Chi instruction. He told us that all top Tai Chi masters practice Chi Gung, specifically, standing Chi Gung.

He said, "Standing Chi Gung develops internal chi and strength like nothing else, like no other practice. You can be a great Tai Chi practitioner without Chi Gung, but with Chi Gung you would become a 'chi filled' and powerful Tai Chi practitioner."

This declaration stuck with me. I continued to include Chi Gung practice with my Tai Chi and also began to develop a separate exploration of Chi Gung exercises. The resulting transformation in my body was profound. I developed deeper relaxation, an increase in the 'softness' that is much talked about in the Internal Martial Arts, and a greater sensitivity and awareness of my body.

After the first two or three years of practicing Chi Gung and Tai Chi, I was so enthusiastic about learning that it affected my whole life. In fact I was so enthusiastic that I did something I had never done before. I built a patio!

Our house in North London at that time had an eighty foot garden. So I thought, "wouldn't it be great if I could practice at the end of the garden where it is quiet and peaceful". The problem was that the end of the garden was a neglected patch of dirt and weeds. Not seeing this as an obstacle, I said to myself "I know, I'll lay down a patio". I was always a bit of a handyman but never saw myself as a builder, thinking that "only builders can lay patios!"

So late one Friday afternoon in the summer of 1990 I began busily digging up the weeds and levelling the dirt. I decided to have light green flagstones with strategically placed red ones on the 20' x10' area I had marked out at the bottom of the garden. The following day I bought and collected bags of sand and ordered the flagstones, which were delivered the same day. I spread a thick layer of sand over the whole area, made a drawing of the pattern I wanted with the flagstones and then began working out from one corner. Laying a stone, checking it for level, putting sand underneath where needed, tamping it down with a large piece of timber and then checking for level again. On about my fifth stone, my neighbour stuck his head over the hedge between our gardens and said, "You need to mix some cement with that sand, otherwise the flagstones will move and sink down". Glad to have some support and guidance, "Oh ok", I said. "I'll do that".

The magic of self awareness

I dashed off, bought some cement and found out what proportions I needed to use. Came back, mixed a batch of cement and sand (I was told that the moisture in the sand and in the air would 'set it off', just enough to make it a firmer foundation) and after re-laying the first five flagstones, continued to lay the rest of them. By darkness I was three quarters of the way finished. Totally pleased with myself, I could not wait to continue my project. I started early next morning and by Sunday afternoon my patio was complete!

Here I stood, on my patio, surveying all before me like a king overseeing his land. I practiced my Standing Chi Gung exercises. My mind became still and I felt like I was in paradise. I could feel the gentle warmth of the day; I could hear the birds singing and also sense the stillness of nature at the bottom of my garden.

However, about a week later, as I practised my standing Chi Gung, bliss was already beginning to fade and I noticed that I had begun to criticize myself, find things wrong with what I was doing, and judge myself harshly. Staying aware of the judgements I was making about myself, I journeyed back to my early years, remembering when my mother used to criticize me for the slightest little thing that I did. Standing in the static Chi Gung postures allowed thoughts and feelings to come to the surface as if fresh and new. This allowed me to see them for what they were, experiences from the past that I had made life determining decisions about. Seeing them clearly allowed them to evaporate from my mind.

This is one of the many benefits of Standing Chi Gung which can take place through the 'magic' of self awareness.

In my early years of learning Tai Chi and Chi Gung, I was told that both of these disciplines were Body-Mind activities. I could not disagree with this in theory, but the reality was, I experienced them both very much as physical exercise........as a beginner I could not do it any other way.

I then came across a book by the successful American gymnast, Dan Millman, called "The Warrior Athlete". At that time, it was always refreshing to read a book by any western person who had different approaches to physical training. A lot of what Dan recounted resonated with my early approach to physical training.

The following 3 pages are extracted from his book.

"For fifteen years I trained with great energy in the sport of gymnastics. In order to succeed (and even survive) I had to develop every conceivable athletic quality, including strength, suppleness, speed of reflexes, stamina, coordination, agility, balance, and a kinesthetic sense, as well as psychological qualities of courage, intense concentration, and serenity.
No matter how hard I applied myself, the process of learning seemed intolerably slow and frustrating. I just couldn't accept the random, haphazard way I learned. Eventually I began to study the process of learning.
Beginning with standard psychological theory, I read every current study of motivation, reinforcement, and learning I could lay my hands on. My understanding grew, but only in bits and pieces. Extensive reading of Eastern philosophy opened up new perspectives, but still the puzzle remained. Then I abandoned experts, theories, and books—and turned to my own intuition."

"I remembered the fact that infants learn at a remarkable pace compared to adults. I began then to watch my little daughter at play, to see if I couldn't discover what qualities she possessed that most adults lacked. Early one Sunday morning I was watching Holly play with the cat on the kitchen floor. My eyes darted from Holly to the cat and back again. Just then, a vision began to crystallize; an intuition was forming about the development of talent—not just physical talent, but emotional and mental talent as well."

"I had noticed that Holly's approach to play was as relaxed and mindless as the cat's. I realized that the essence of talent is not so much the presence of certain qualities, but rather the absence of self and society-imposed obstructions. Young children appear to be free of the mental, physical, and emotional obstructions which we unconsciously develop in our later years."

"After that discovery, I decided that if there were any ultimate clues to be found, they would appear in the pre-civilized world of nature. I found myself taking long walks alone, observing the natural forces and their relationship to the creatures and vegetation and to the earth. At first, I only skimmed the surface, recording the obvious— that plants tend to grow toward the sun, that objects fall toward the earth and rivers flow downhill. These were elementary-school observations; yet I didn't know how else to begin."

"After many such walks, my vision cleared. Nature removed her veil, and I was able to see her lessons. I saw trees bending in the wind, and understood the principle of nonresistance. Visualizing how gentle running water can cut through solid rock, I grasped the law of accommodation. Seeing how all living things thrived in moderate cycles, I was able to understand the principle of balance. Observing the regular passing of the seasons, each coming in its own good time, taught me the natural order of life."

"I realized that I had become alienated from the natural

pattern, but that my daughter still knew no separation from things as they are. After all my searching, these insights were a delight to me—and gave new meaning to athletic training. Still, it all seemed more poetical than practical. . . until, all in a single moment, the final piece fell into place.

I was taking a warm shower, enjoying the soothing spray. My thoughts were quiet; then out of nowhere, a realization came and left me stunned: "The laws are psychophysical!" This may not seem like a great realization to you, but I dropped the soap."

"Realizing that nature's laws applied equally to the human psyche, inseparable from the human body, made all the difference for me. With that the world turned upside down. No longer would I view the principles of my training as merely physical in their implications. From that day on, athletic training was to become a psychophysical challenge. The world no longer seemed just a static physical object. Now it was filled with energy and movement and subtle things. This episode reconnected my psyche to the universal laws, and reaffirmed my essential participation in nature."

"All that remained was to put this understanding to use—to apply it fully to a new way of athletic training. Through such training we could all re-awaken our innate ability to learn, and our athletic development would inevitably spill over into our daily lives. For the first time, I really saw the relevance of athletics, and saw how training could become a meaningful way of life.

The game of athletics expanded beyond physical fitness, recreation, or entertainment; it had become a perfect model for the Game of Life."

So as I continued to develop, I began to teach. With my teaching, I became that purist I mentioned earlier. That is, I would not compromise the standards I set myself. I would not compromise the teaching standards that I had been trained in and strongly believe in. What that meant, is that the style of teaching that I was adhering to strictly, is the traditional way of teaching i.e. personally demonstrating, thus passing on information and transmitting what I knew. I ensured that everyone I taught had personal attention using one to one and small group teaching methods.

This served me well, as I attracted like minded people who had similar goals and standards, thus teaching became personally challenging and very enjoyable. My students enjoyed my light and humorous approach, which embodies the qualities of focus and dedication to practice ……"for what you practice you surely become"

However, those who wanted a softer approach were excluded from having an ongoing experience of the benefits of the amazing art of Chi Gung. For example, some people would come to my classes or events and comment that my approach to Chi Gung was simply a 'bit too intense'.

For many years my students have encouraged me to show more people what Chi Gung can do, and I have found a perfect solution for those who want a gentler and softer practice. So for about 7 years I have been able to include people of all abilities and conditions through the Shibashi set of Chi Gung exercises. These exercises are the perfect way for people to learn how to relax while being active, to cultivate the feeling sense of meditation and to experience the flow of natural life force through their bodies, and become more fluid and flexible while enjoying movement to music.

Recently, I decided that I shouldn't shy away from what's been in the back of my mind – to integrate technology of the 21st century. This would enable me to teach online, sell DVDs, and upload videos, share MP3 files and much more. In this way I can share what I know with as many people as possible.

What is in my heart, is for as many people as possible to benefit from this ancient art, so needed to balance our modern lifestyle. Yes, I want to continue to build it as a profitable business as well, and be rewarded for my long years of study and committed hard work.

For many years I resisted the softer styles of Chi Gung, thinking that they were inferior to traditional Yang style Tai Chi, which I had been learning for many years. What I failed to recognise, was that all good Tai Chi practice, as well as good Chi Gung practice, enabled you to attain softness in your body – without weakness.

What I would like to pass on now is that as your practice continues, whether it is Tai Chi or Chi Gung, you must ongoingly develop softness. This increases sensitivity in your body, allows joints to open up and nurtures the kinaesthetic sense i.e. the awareness of the position and movement of the parts of the body.

My journey with Chi Gung continues. From its beginnings more than 25 years ago I have found it to be a great ally in my life. Freeing me from stress, helping me to calm my mind and allowing me to appreciate the genuine beauty that is life itself……..pretty good results from moving, breathing and focused attention!

People have their 'realizations' in different ways. Some have the 'epiphany' moment and others gain their insights through patience and persistence. I tend to get mine with the latter.

Through my persistence with Chi Gung exercises I have seen that this form of exercise can benefit so many people. The principles are simple and easy to apply. Simply apply them in your practice!

I've worked on the Shibashi set of Chi Gung movements in such a way that that they are now easy to follow, easy to do and easy to understand. Most people FEEL the results very quickly.

The unique Shibashi exercises are a set of 18 movements, designed to enhance the flow of energy in your body and thus improve your well-being and enjoyment of life. To this day I keep refining what I learn, so that people who learn from me can start from scratch and begin to reap the benefits of a system that will transform positively their state of stress. Thanks to the technology available today on the internet, I am able to:

- follow my passion of sharing what I've learnt with as many people as possible
- make videos of what I know, you can download them or view them online
- make valuable information available – all you need is a computer/laptop and an internet connection
- produce DVDs that you can purchase www.taichiteambuilding.co.uk
- give you advice no matter where you are, or I am, in the world. We truly have become a global village
- communicate in real time, so if we choose we can see each other and speak at the same time, for example Skype

Consistently throughout the past 25 years, I have built my knowledge and gained expertise in the basics as well as the so called 'secrets' of internal alchemy– which for beginners means:-

- How to focus your mind
- How to use the correct rhythm of breathing
- How to move in such a way that you actually generate energy rather than expend energy

Putting these three fundamental principles together has enabled me to teach a system that REALLY works from the moment you start using it.

These special types of exercises are for building natural inner strength and enhancing your well being by harnessing the most powerful health creating tool the world has ever known – Chi Gung.

What's more, it doesn't matter what age or level of fitness you have, because Chi Gung, sometimes called the new science of the 21st century, will ALWAYS work………as long as you practice the tried and tested principles.

Chapter 2

What is Chi Gung?

"Do the difficult things while they are easy and do the great things while they are small. A journey of a thousand miles must begin with a single step." Lao Tzu

These days many people already know something about *Qigong*. It is now popular around the world.

Qigong is an ancient Chinese practice that works to make us healthier. *Qi* (pronounced `chee') means vital energy; *Gong* means work. So *Qigong* is an exercise that works on our vital energy. Vital energy is our life force and without it we cannot survive. *Qigong* is a way to make us healthier and allow us to live longer by creating extra *Qi* in the body to make the *Qi* we were born with stronger. *Qigong* is also a way of guiding our own healing and bringing our body back into harmony with nature.

There are many countries and cultures that have their own ways of working with *Qi* or vital energy. However, what makes *Qigong* different from others is that it is based on the principles of Traditional Chinese Medicine (TCM), which is, in turn, based upon the understanding of the Yin/Yang and Five Element theory, acupuncture points, meridians and the Dantian (the centre of our body, where *Qi* is stored). This knowledge is only found in TCM and in Chinese martial arts. This is why *Qigong* is a Chinese skill.

There are many different styles of *Qigong*, originating from five schools of thought: Daoism, Buddhism, Confucianism, martial and medical (healing). However, all have the same principle of making the vital energy stronger and the body healthy.

Qigong dates back over 3,000 years. During this time, ancient Chinese people lived along the Yellow River, and they had to find ways to survive in that area. As there was a lot of water there and often flooding, the climate was very damp. The people suffered a lot of problems with their joints, like arthritis and rheumatism, because the damp got inside their bodies. It is the same today in many colder countries, such as Britain, Canada, Russia and the north of China. When the damp gets inside the body, it tends to stay in the joints, just like the dust in your house collects in the corners where it is difficult to clean.

These ancient people had to find a way to live in their damp environment, but what could they do? They found the best way was the same as cleaning the dust from our clothes or rugs: to shake them clean. But how do we shake the body? It is easy. All we have to do is move. The ancient Chinese created many different kinds of movements, some of which were like a dance and others which were based upon observations from nature and movements from animals.

These movements might have started in the same way as Polynesians, Africans and Australian Aborigines created their own cultural dances. However, whereas these cultures danced to commune with nature or tell a story, the movements that these peoples created were particularly for health. These peoples had their own ways to move the body to create internal heat in order to clear dampness and illnesses. This has been documented through old drawings found on bronze vessels and on silk.

Qigong is good for more than getting rid of damp in the joints, however. It helps to balance the body and alleviates all kinds of conditions such as stomach ache, poor circulation, backache, headaches and so on. It releases negative energy and stiffness, so when the ancient Chinese people moved in this special way, they felt lighter and happier and had more energy.

Q*igong* practice also needs balance. I have come across many people who do a lot of movement but no meditation. They end up sustaining injuries, particularly in their joints. Some people, on the other hand, do a lot of meditation and no movement, but this makes their bodies weak and they do not have enough strength to get through the day easily. For our health to stay balanced, we need both the movement and meditation. This covers both Yin and Yang and will make us healthy.

Practicing Chi Gung correctly will assist you to create positive energy in your life. Positive energy is not a hyped-adrenaline-rush type of energy. It is a carefully nurtured expression of your natural state of being.

The Way of Energy

The goal of Chi Kung exercise is to stimulate the flow of energy internally in the body so that it effectively rushes through and clears the entire network of Chi channels, or "meridians".

Extensive research has been done over the years to develop a system of exercise that would speed up the blood circulation (and hence also stimulate the flow of Chi) without placing an intolerable strain on the lungs. The results drew on the accumulated wisdom of Chinese Taoist and Buddhist breathing practices and the practices and disciplines of the martial arts. Chi Kung, as the resulting exercises were known, used a series of breathing exercises to control the internal movement of Chi while the body remained virtually motionless.

For centuries most knowledge about Chi Kung was passed on within families or small circles of masters and students and kept relatively secret. It is only recently that it has been taught and discussed publicly. There are a growing number of applications of Chi Kung exercise, ranging from the treatment of chronic illness through to the development of extraordinary physical powers that enable practitioners to break stones with their bare fingers. Now, it is increasingly being used to assist in the treatment of illnesses that Western medical practice cannot treat successfully. It is also being used to help prevent illness by building up the body's immune systems and internal strength. What Chi Kung offers is a method of training the nervous system, the mind, and the internal organs simultaneously, so that the inner strength of the whole person is raised to a new level of power and fitness.

ONE DESTINATION, MANY ROUTES

There are many styles and schools of Chi Kung. There is Chi Kung for health, therapy, martial arts and spiritual development. There are Buddhist and Taoist schools of Chi Kung.

In athletics Chi Kung is used to develop muscle power and endurance. In medicine, especially in China, there are two main branches of Chi Kung: one is moving Chi Kung which involves movement and exercise; the other is limited to static breathing and meditational exercises.

In the martial arts, Chi Kung training includes techniques known as "iron palm", "iron shirt", and "metal bell cover".

In the spiritual field, there are Chi Kung exercises that enable the student to experience other dimensions, and to develop telepathic powers.

The goal, however, of building internal strength, remains fundamental to all.

STATIC CHI GUNG–ZHANZHUANG–STANDING LIKE A TREE

The ability to transform energy and even create it within you is one of the profound secrets of life. Like a tree, you are one of the great power-stations of nature. You share a deep affinity with the countless trees and saplings that surround you on the planet. They have much to teach us. They are perfectly adapted to the rhythm of the seasons. They combine immense strength with the most delicate sensitivity. They turn sunlight and

air into fuel. They share the earth with others, but are secure within themselves.
This is the vision of life so beautifully expressed in the ancient Taoist classic of Lao Tzu, the Tao Teh Ching:

Standing alone and unchanging,
One can observe every mystery,
Present at every moment and ceaselessly continuing
This is the gateway to
indescribable marvels.

This is one of the earliest references to Zhan Zhuang. You are standing like a tree, alone and unmoving. You come to understand everything that happens within you — all the internal changes that take place in your organs and muscles. You practise constantly. You feel the reactions taking place. The feeling never stops. It goes on and on, over and over again. This is the Way: no matter how far you go you will never come to the end of all the wondrous things there are to discover.

The Remainder of this chapter is extracted from a book following a personal journey about learning Chen style Tai Chi and Chi Gung by someone called Kinthessa. The book is called –'Turning Silk'.

The practice of ZhanZhuang. This standing *Qigong* instills the capacity to listen to one's body and learn to see its energetic workings. The practice took root in us, day by day, on this and subsequent visits to Sydney. At the beginning, the adjustments were gross, and grew finer as our bodies became more aligned, as we became more sensitive to the connection between posture and *Qi* flow.

One of the surprises in store for the person who takes to regular standing practice is the ease with which the raised arms may be maintained. When one is first introduced to ZhanZhuang, it is natural to worry that standing unmoving for a stretch of time will be uncomfortable; the additional thought, that the arms are to be held raised up for the whole time, can be quite alarming. Of course there will be aches and fatigue to begin with, but much of the difficulty is simply the result of tension.

We are used to holding ourselves up by our chests, necks and shoulders. There is tremendous effort involved in this daily practice that we all do unwittingly! When we decide we want to live differently, we can begin to change our habits. The mind can learn to let go of the body. There is no need to hang on to our arms. We may find that standing with arms up is easier than standing with the arms down. The arms can support the stance, they provide an ample surround for the body. These days, when my shoulders or neck feel tired, I stand, and this cures me of aches and pains. It is a great relief to earth the body.

When you see someone stock-still with the eyes closed, apparently oblivious of their surroundings, it looks kind of strange. When Ben's sister comes in upon one or both of us in ZhanZhuang, she says, "Oh, you're standing like a tree!" Even though she is an acupuncturist of thirty years' experience she is a little surprised.

There are myriad things on the move. Standing still makes one keenly aware of them. The whole body is a mass of buzzings. Some are collected in bunches, while others are like fireflies flashing in the night. It is not dark inside. In a sense, the eye is looking and seeing what is going on, it has learned "to look more closely, not at things but at a world closer to myself, looking from an inner place to one further within." One also hears, with which sense I could not say. The entire body is listening to itself. The calmer the mind is, the deeper the sensing.

My favourite time of the year for ZhanZhuang practice is winter. Here in the valley, the silence can fall so thickly that it absorbs all disturbances. Attachments to other places loosen and I feel myself adrift on the surface of a vast stillness.

It is good to be cold when starting practice. Our house has no central heating, and the winters are old-fashioned ones, the heat coming from the cooking stove in the kitchen, and the wood stove in the den. When I begin ZhanZhuang in this season, I can follow better the flow of *Qi* as it quickens in the cold body. First there is the sensation of tiny tricklings, like water oozing out of crevices in the body here and there. It is usually a warm sensation, but it can also be a delicious tingling which is almost cool. As isolated areas link up, a tracery of pathways begins to appear; I call them pathways, for they have direction and continuity. Once the standing gets under way, the acute stirrings against the background of chill in the body become generalized, and I can feel as warm as toast.

Now we are enjoying some mild February days. I have come to appreciate this month's place in the scheme of things; there is much afoot in this period. I have been taking the chance to be outside. I regret that this book cannot include the sound of the birds calling, and the swishing of the wind.

In ZhanZhuang, changes happen both of their own accord and because you make them happen. When you become an adept in the practice, these two ways are often one: your guidance of the process is so fine that there is no doing as such, it is 'Doing Nothing'. This is not a distant goal if you practise regularly. You begin by observing things as they are; you notice tension here and there, pulls this way and that. There is a way to approach the matter where you leave distance between what you observe and yourself.

Much can be moved simply by breathing and awareness. Tension begins to dissolve around a joint, for example, giving more room for maneuvering it into a better alignment. Such changes are guided not so much by effort as by intent. On the other hand there are moments, e.g. when I try to alter the hip and leg alignment by specific and effortful moves. Each alteration like this needs to be given time.

There is the action, then a phase of staying with what is happening, when you do nothing except observe; with care, you do not move. These phases are where you see *Qi* at work. A certain adjustment, the tinier the more powerful when you become attuned to the practice, brings about shifts throughout your body. It is essential that you do not interfere with them. A joint is held together, for better or worse, by many connected threads, too many to separate out. Reorganizing a joint affects all these threads. Let one alteration sort itself out for a good while; this is the best way to proceed.

And what does it mean, this sorting out by itself? The *Qi*, as delicate as it is, is an effective force. We cannot see it concretely, but given time and calm, its activity is discernible. When a habitual holding around a joint, for example, is momentarily released, the surrounding area absorbs the initial change. From here emanate shifts further and further afield. We can talk about this in terms of physical parts, these days more and more finely separated out, although most likely, we cannot feel them individually. But what we do experience is the spreading of warmth, a cool tingling, a sense of inward expansion, an aeration, the feelings of a pleasant flowing; or sometimes seemingly the opposite, an increase in density, even a startling shift, a kind of jolting into place. In any case, a lot of sensations hard to define but definitely on the move. These are some of the manifestations of *Qi*. With further release of habitual tensions, longer and longer phases of allowing a stirring to waft about, a new body is slowly built. An energetic body.

I finish this account as the southwestern hills deepen into blue greys, the sky above them tinged apricot.

Bare attention, an incisive awareness, are the tools one needs for deepening ZhanZhuang practice. Attention moves through the body like the knife of Zhuangzi's Cook Ting* (see below). Breathing becomes very soft and barely there. A deep silence penetrates, even as one feels oneself being slowly kneaded and pulped.

*Cook Ting was cutting up an ox for Lord Wen-hui. As every touch of his hand, every heave of his shoulder, every move of his feet, every thrust of his knee — zip! zoop! He slithered the knife along with a zing, and all was in perfect rhythm, as though he were performing the dance of the Mulberry Grove or keeping time to the Ching-shou music.

"Ah, this is marvellous!" said Lord Wen-hui. "Imagine skill reaching such heights!"

Cook Ting laid down his knife and replied, "What I care about is the Way, which goes beyond skill. When I first began cutting up oxen, all I could see was the ox itself. After three years I no longer saw the whole ox. And now — now I go at it by spirit and don't look with my eyes. Perception and understanding have come to a stop and spirit moves where it wants. I go along with the natural makeup, strike in the big hollows, guide the knife through the big openings, and following things as they are. So I never touch the smallest ligament or tendon, much less a main joint."

"A good cook changes his knife once a year — because he cuts. A mediocre cook changes his knife once a month — because he hacks. I've had this knife of mine for nineteen years and I've cut up thousands of oxen with it, and yet the blade is as good as though it had just come from the grindstone. There are spaces between the joints, and the blade of the knife has really no thickness. If you insert what has no thickness into such spaces, then there's plenty of room — more than enough for the blade to play about it. That's why after nineteen years the blade of my knife is still as good as when it first came from the grindstone."

"However, whenever I come to a complicated place, I size up the difficulties, tell myself to watch out and be careful, keep my eyes on what I'm doing, work very slowly, and move the knife with the greatest subtlety, until — flop! the whole thing comes apart like a clod of earth crumbling to the ground. I stand there holding the knife and look all around me, completely satisfied and reluctant to move on, and then I wipe off the knife and put it away."

"Excellent!" said Lord Wen-hui. "I have heard the words of Cook Ting and learned how to care for life!"

Translated by Burton Watson (Chuang Tzu: The Basic Writings, 1964)

Chapter 3

An Overview of Chi Gung

*– extracted from 'Opening the Energy Gates'
by Bruce Kumar Frantzis*

Traditionally in China, the main schools of Chi Kung emphasized maintaining health and preventing disease. They believed that many illnesses are caused by mental and emotional excesses. When a person's mind is not calm, balanced, and peaceful, the organs will not function normally. For example, depression can cause stomach ulcers and indigestion. Anger will cause the liver to malfunction. Sadness will cause stagnation and tightness in the lungs, and fear can disturb the normal functioning of the kidneys and bladder. They realized that if you want to avoid illness, you must learn to balance and relax your thoughts and emotions. This is called "regulating the mind."

In order to reach the goal of a calm and peaceful mind, their training focused on regulating the mind, body, and breath. They believed that as long as these three things were regulated, the Chi flow would be smooth and sickness would not occur. This is called "Shiou Chi," which means "cultivating Chi." Shiou in Chinese means to regulate, to cultivate, or to repair. It means to maintain in good condition. This is very different from the Taoist Chi training after the Han dynasty which was called "Liann Chi," which is translated "train Chi." Liann means to drill or to practice to make stronger.

Chi and Man

In order to use Chi Kung to maintain and improve your health, you must know that there is Chi in your body, and you must understand how it circulates and what you can do to insure that the circulation is smooth and strong.

Chi is energy. It is a requirement for life. The Chi in your body cannot be seen, but it can be felt. This Chi can make your body feel too positive (too Yang) or too negative (too Yin).

Imagine that your physical body is a machine, and your Chi is the current that makes it run. Without the current the machine is dead and unable to function. For example, when you pinch yourself, you feel pain. Have you ever thought "how do I feel pain?" You might answer that it is because you have a nervous system in your body which perceives the pinch and sends a signal to the brain.

However, there is more to it than that. The nervous system is material, and if it didn't have energy circulating in it, it wouldn't function. Chi is the energy which makes the nervous system and the other parts of your body work. When you pinch your skin, that area is stimulated and the chi field is disturbed. Your brain is designed to sense this and other disturbances, and to interpret the cause.

Chinese Chi Kung has started to bloom in the West. More and more, people are coming to believe that in addition to maintaining health and increasing longevity, Chi Kung can be one of the most effective ways to attain a peaceful, spiritual life.

Chi Kung is one of the greatest achievements of China. It was created from the accumulated experiences of countless generations by thousands of "wise men." These wise men, after learning the traditional knowledge, modified and added their own experiences to the practice. Finally, this treasure has reached our hands. Now, it is our responsibility to keep it and continue to develop it.

Many of the theories and training methods of Chi Kung were kept secret, and only recently made available to the general public.

There are many reasons for this secrecy:

1. Every Chi Kung style considered its theory and methods to be precious treasures which offered something which could not be purchased with money, namely health and long life. Because this was so valuable many masters did not want to share it.

2. Many Chi Kung training theories are hard to understand, and the practices dangerous if done incorrectly. Only advanced students have the necessary level of understanding, and few ever get to this level.
3. Many Chi Kung practitioners believed that the more you kept a mystery, the more valuable and precious it would be.

4. Some of the Chi Kung training, such as Marrow/Brain Washing, involves stimulation of the sexual organs. In the ancient, conservative society, this was considered immoral.

Many Chi Kung secrets were passed down only to a few students or to direct blood relatives. In religious Chi Kung, the limitations were even stricter. The religious exercises were passed down only to the priests. This was especially true for the Marrow/Brain Washing Chi Kung. In fact, these techniques were traditionally passed down to only a very few disciples who understood Chi Kung theory and had reached a high level of cultivation. This situation lasted until the beginning of the 20th century, when it was gradually revealed to laymen. It was only during the last forty years that many of the secret documents were made available to the public.

Nobody can deny that Western science which has been developed today is mainly focused on material development. Spiritual science has been downplayed. The major reason for this is simply that the spiritual energy world is harder to see and understand. This spiritual science is still in its formative stage.

Recently, it was reported that even today's science understands probably only 10% of the functions of the human brain. You can see from this, that compared to the 'great nature" which is still waiting for us to discover and understand it, science today is still in its infancy.

For these reasons, it is unwise to use today's infant science to judge the accumulated experience and phenomena of the past. I believe that as long as we respect the traditions and experience of the past, and continue our study and research, we will eventually be able to understand all of these natural phenomena scientifically.

Following this reasoning, traditional Chi Kung theory and training methods should remain the main source and authority for your training. The correct attitude in practicing Chi Kung is to respect and understand the past, and to also examine everything from a modern, scientific point of view. In this way you can improve upon the knowledge and experience of the past. The "secrets" should be opened to the public and should accept the questioning of modern science. A secret is a secret only if you do not know it. Once a secret is common knowledge, then it ceases to be a secret.

People who exercise a lot and whose bodies are externally strong are not necessarily healthier or happier than the average person. In order to have true good health you must have a healthy body, a healthy mind, and also smooth and balanced Chi circulation.

According to Chinese medicine, many illnesses are caused by imbalances in your mind. For example, worry and nervousness can upset your stomach or harm your spleen. Fear or fright can hinder the normal functioning of your kidneys and bladder. This is because your internal energy (Chi circulation) is closely related to your mind. In order to be truly healthy, you must have both a healthy physical body and a calm and healthy mind. True good health is both external and internal.

In order to have a long life, you need to have not only a healthy physical body and smooth Chi circulation, but also training in two more disciplines. The first concerns your blood, the second your spirit. Your blood runs through your entire body. If your blood cells are not healthy, it does not matter how healthy and strong your physical body and organs appear to be, because your physical body will degenerate quickly. The marrow is the factory which makes your blood cells. If you know how to keep your marrow healthy and fresh, the quality of the blood cells will be high. When these healthy and fresh blood cells are running in your physical body, the degeneration process will slow down and your lifespan will increase.

The Background of Chi Gung

There are five major branches of Chi Gung in China: Taoist, Buddhist, medical, martial arts, and Confucian. The original Chi Gung was Taoist, which was the source for the others. The Taoist form created Chinese medicine over 4000 years ago, discovering the points and meridian lines of acupuncture and the medicinal uses of thousands of herbs.

Taoist Chi Gung equally emphasizes cultivating physical vitality and developing spirit or consciousness through meditation. It seeks long life with vibrant health into old age, as well as a living spiritual awareness that manifests daily here and now, not in an afterlife. In contrast, Buddhist Chi Gung focuses more on the health of the soul than that of the body.

The other three branches of Chi Gung borrowed techniques from both the Taoists and Buddhists, and recombined them for specific purposes. For example, the Confucians stress applying Chi Gung to intellectual or aesthetic practices, such as painting or calligraphy; medical Chi Gung utilizes chi to cure disease, relieve pain, heal injuries, and maintain ongoing wellness; martial arts Chi Gung seeks to create exceptional physical abilities and psychic awareness.

How Chi Gung Is Practiced

All Chi Gung exercises are performed in a relaxed, gentle fashion that does not cause shock to the body All stretches must be done to only 70 percent of capacity not 100 percent. Chi Gung exercises are the most effective and sophisticated low impact exercises that have ever existed. Chi Gung does not build dynamic muscles; rather, it uses breathing, stretching, movement, and visualization to develop chi, a strong functional body, and a calm and relaxed mind. Through practice, the joints, internal organs, and glands are all strengthened. The Chi Gung approach to exercise is thus radically different from the typical Western approach. In my 30 years of experience in the martial arts and in Oriental healing I saw at least a thousand practitioners of Chi Gung who were as relaxed, flexible, and capable at the age of eighty as is the average twenty to thirty year old.

The fundamental methodology of Chi Gung involves the use of the chi to activate the body's internal pumping mechanisms for the purpose of moving bodily fluids more efficiently Chi Gung exercises are, in effect, the energetic equivalent of pumping iron.

The body, being mostly fluids, has several internal pumping mechanisms besides the cardiovascular system (the cerebrospinal system, for example).

Chi Gung works by increasing the flow of chi to these internal pumps. Blood, which carries oxygen and nutrients to the body's cells and removes their waste products, is perhaps the most important body fluid. Chi Gung has methods for moving blood through the veins and arteries just as strongly as does Western style aerobics, but without strain. Rather than solely emphasizing cardiovascular pulmonary exercises, Chi Gung contains specialized motions for the liver, kidneys, spleen, and various glands and nerves.

Chi Gung may be practiced standing still, moving, sitting, or lying down. Of the many Chi Gung systems in China, the one probably most familiar to the West is Tai Chi Chuan, but many of the exercises (such as the Eight Pieces of Brocade, the Five Animal Play, and the Yi Jin Jing) are equally well known in China, where Chi Gung is now enjoying a revival, with 60 to 70 million followers.

Most Chinese who practice do so to be vibrantly healthy or to cure specific diseases; many who practice are older people who are experiencing the realities of aging and want to do something about it. While in some regions Chi Gung is taking on the character of a revivalist religious movement (with healing through the laying on of hands), simultaneously whole clinics, hospitals, and exercise centres are being devoted to advancing the health benefits of Chi Gung from a scientific point of view.

The computer revolution has become possible because ways have been found to pass electricity between all parts of the computer hardware with greater and greater efficiency. The Chinese have long recognized that, by increasing and balancing the power of the chi in the body, a similar positive revolution can occur within the individual. Currently, Chi Gung represents a new frontier in Western medicine. As time passes, and the concepts and principles of Chi Gung become understood in Western terms, this ancient way of keeping fit will bring health benefits throughout the Western Hemisphere. That, least, is my fervent hope.

Kumar Frantzis,
Fairfax, California

Chapter 4

Some Chi Gung History

"A leader is best when people barely know he exists, when his work is done, his aim fulfilled, they will say: we did it ourselves." Lao Tzu

The Development of *Qigong*

Qigong, as an art of healing and health preservation, is thought to have originated as early as four thousand years ago in the *Tang Yao* times, as a form of dancing.

Lu's Spring and Autumn Annals or Lu's History (Lu Shi Chun Qiu) records, in the beginning of the Tao Tang Tribes, the sun was often shut off by heavy clouds and it rained all the time; turbulent waters overflowed the rivers' banks. People lived a gloomy and dull life and suffered from rigidity of their joints.

As a remedy dancing was recommended. From the experience of their long-term struggle with nature, the ancients gradually realized that body movements, exclamations and various ways of breathing could help readjust certain bodily functions. For example, imitating animal movements such as climbing, looking about, and leaping was found to promote a vital flow of *Qi*.

Pronouncing "Hi" was found to either decrease or increase strength, "Ha" could disperse heat, and "Xu" could alleviate pain. In this way, *Qigong* was brought into being.

During the Spring and Autumn and the Warring States

Periods (770-221 b.c.), various schools of thought arose. Such schools rationalized and raised to the level of theory, their knowledge of nature, society and life, based on the experiences of their predecessors. Through this process, *Qigong* found its way to systematization and became an independent theoretical construct popular with philosophers and scholars.

The theories of *Qigong* continued to develop and coalesce into powerful new concepts such as the three treasures of the human body (life essence, *Qi*, and mental faculties). *Qigong* methods also started to develop during this time. "Exhale and inhale to expel the stale and take in the fresh", "a bear twists its neck", or "a bird stretches its wings," are a few examples of such methods.

The Qin (221-207 B.C.) and Han (206 B. C.-A.D. 220) dynasties saw a rapid development of medical skills, which in turn enhanced *Qigong* theory and practice. *The Yellow Emperor's Canon of Internal Medicine*, the earliest medical classic extant in China, described Daoyin, Guidance of *Qi*, and An Qiao as important curative measures that could also preserve life. It also offered the following advice, which besides offering a general life philosophy, describes the state of mind necessary for successful *Qigong* practice:
"Be indifferent to fame or gain, be alone in repose, and take the various parts of the body as an organic whole."

There is an account of *Daoyin* found in *Plain Questions on Acupuncture (Su Wen Yi Pian Ci Fa Lun)* that says,

"Patients with lingering kidney disease may face south from 3 to 5 A.M., concentrate the mind, hold back the breath, crane the neck and swallow *Qi* as if swallowing a hard object seven times. After that, there would be a great amount of fluid welling up from under the tongue." In 1973, a silk book, *Fasting and Taking Qi (Que Gu Shi Qi Pian)* and a silk painting *Daoyin Chart (Dao Yin Tu)* of the Western Han dynasty (206 B.C.-A.D. 24) were unearthed from the Han Dynasty Tomb Mawangdui No. 3 in Changsha, Hunan Province. The book records the *Daoyin* method for guiding *Qi* and the chart covers 44 colored paintings presenting human figures imitating the movements of a wolf, monkey, ape, bear, crane, hawk, and vulture.

Thus, they reveal that the Chinese began to teach *Qigong* pictorially as early as the beginning of the Western Han dynasty. The two outstanding medical scholars Zhang Zhongjing and Hua Tuo, in the closing years of the Eastern Han dynasty (A.D. 25-220), both aided in the development of *Qigong*.

In his great work, *Synopsis of the Prescriptions of the Golden Chamber Yin Kui Yao Luo)*, Zhang Zhongiing stated that "As soon as heaviness and sluggishness of the extremities is felt, start Daoyin, breathing exercises, acupuncture, moxibustion, and massage with application of ointment to prevent obstruction of the nine orifices." The famous exercise Frolics of Five Animals (*Wu Qin Xi*) was devised during this time by Hua Tuo and became widely practiced and it is still popular today.

During the Wei dynasty (A.D. 220-265), the Jin dynasty (A.D. 265-420), and the Northern and Southern dynasties (A.D. 420-589), *Qigong* developed as a way of preserving health and as a method for treating disease through the emission of *Qi*. Zhang Zhan of the Jin dynasty listed in his work *Yang Sheng Essentials of Health Preservation (Yao Ji)* ten essential practices, of which thrifty of mentality, preservation of *Qi*, conservation of constitution, and *Daoyin* were all related to *Qigong*. Tao Hongjing of the Northern and Southern dynasties recorded in his book, *Health Preservation and Longevity (Yang Sheng Yan Ming Lu)*, many ancient *Qigong* methods and theories.

In *The History of the Jin Dynasty yin Shu)*, there is an account of doctor Xing Ling who became famous for using outgoing *Qi* to cure a patient who had suffered more than ten years from flaccidity arthralgia syndrome. As a result of this success, many more people became interested in medical *Qigong*.

Qigong was widely put into clinical application in the Sui (A.D. 581-618) the Tang (A.D. 618-907) dynasties. The books *General Treatise on the Causes and Symptoms of Diseases (Zhu Bing Yuan Hou Lun)*, *Prescriptions Worth a Thousand Gold for Emergencies (Bei Ji Qian Jin Yao Fang)* and *The Medical Secrets of Official (Wai Tai Mi Yao)* contain a wealth of *Qigong* therapies for treating specific pathologies.

The General Treatise on the Cause and Symptoms of Diseases, records more than 260 *Qigong* therapies, The *Brahman Method* of Indian Massage and Laozi Massage along with other *Qigong Daoyin* massage methods of health preservation in the text, *Prescriptions Worth a Thousand Gold for Emergencies*. *Master Huan Zhen's Knacks in Taking Qi (Huan Zhen Xian Sheng Fu Nei Zhi Qi Jue)* of the Tang dynasty describes the *Pithy Formulae of Qi Distribution*, which introduces the essential principles and techniques for emitting outgoing *Qi*.

During the period of the Song (A.D. 960-1279), Jin (A.D. 1115— 1234), and Yuan (A.D. 1271-1368) dynasties, an upsurge of Daoist exercises for cultivating spiritual energy *Qigong* began to merge with these exercises giving rise to more sophisticated forms of therapeutic *Qigong*. Within the book *The Complete Record of Holy Benevolence (Sheng Ji Zong Lu)* is a wealth of *Qigong* information. Many *Qigong* descriptions can also be found in the works of the four eminent physicians of the Jin and Yuan dynasties.

Li Dongyuan wrote in his book, *Secret Record of the Chamber of Orchids (Lan Shi Mi Cang)*, "Falling ill, the patient should sit still at ease to replenish *Qi*." Liu Wansu mentioned, in his *Etiology Based on Plain Questions (Su Wen Xuan Ji Bing Yuan Shi)*, the application of the Six Character Formulae in the treatment of diseases.

Zhu Zhenheng stated in his book, *Danxi's Experiential Therapy (Dan Xi Xin Fa)*, that "Patients with syncope, flaccidity, or cold or heat syndrome due to stagnation of *Qi* should be treated with *Daoyin* exercises."

During the period of the Ming (A.D. 1368-1644) and Qing (A.D.1644-1911) dynasties, doctors characterized the development of *Qigong* by deeper mastery and wider application. This enriched the medical books with *Qigong* literature and data. Abundant *Qigong* information was included in several influential books: *A Retrospective Collection of Medical Classics (Yi Jing Su Hui Ji)* by Wang Lu, *Wanmizhai's Ten Categories of Medical Works (Wan Mi Zhai Yi Shu Shi Zhong)* by Wan Quan, and *The General Medicine of the Past and Present (Gu Jin Yi Tong Da Quan)* compiled by Xu Chunpu.

The great physician Li Shizhen stated definitively in his book, *A Study on the Eight Extra Channels (Qi Jing Ba Mai Kao)*, that "The internal conditions and the channels can only be perceived by those who can see things by inward vision." This famous thesis indicated the relationship between *Qigong* and the channels and collaterals.

Qigong has gained higher priority and more rapid development since the founding of the People's Republic of China. In 1955, a *Qigong* hospital was established in Tangshan. During this time two important books introduced exercises such as internal cultivation, keep-fit, and many others, thus, giving an impetus to the development of *Qigong* research throughout the whole country. These books are *The Practice of Qigong Therapy (Liao Fa Shi Jian)* written by Liu Guizhen and *Qigong* and *Keep-fit Qigong (Qi Gong Ji Bao Jian Qi Gong)* written by Hu Yaozhen.

Since 1978, medical workers and *Qigong* masters all over China have made vigorous efforts to popularize *Qigong* for health preservation and disease prevention. Some scientists and technicians have not only studied *Qigong* in terms of physiology, biochemistry and modern medicine, but they have also conducted multi-disciplinary research efforts to analyze the physical effect of outgoing *Qi*.

A study on the nature and essence of *Qigong* has thus been initiated, and *Qigong*, as a new branch of science, has entered a period of vigorous development. *Qigong* research societies, hospitals and departments have been established to research, teach and use *Qigong*. *Qigong* practice and study have become commonplace throughout China.

Since the 1990's many *Qigong* journals and magazines have been published. Journals include: *The Journal of Qigong (Qi Gong Za Zhi), Qigong and Science (Qi Gong Yu Ke Xue), China Qigong (Zhong Hua Qi Gong), Chinese Qigong (Zhong Guo Qi Gong),* and *Orient Qigong (Dong Fang Qi Gong).*

Chapter 5

Modern Teachers

"A true friend is someone who sees the pain in your eyes while everyone else believes the smile on your face." Unknown

There are now many Chi Gung teachers in Europe, the Americas and many other countries around the world. The greatest number of Chi Gung teachers is in the country of origin of these powerful exercises, namely China. One of the greatest legacies given to the world from China is this profound art and science of Chi Gung.

I have learnt from all the teachers I mention in this book. Either directly one to one, in their classes or at their workshops. Some I have learned from via their books or videos.

James Holland

James Holland is also known as San Gee Tam. San Gee Tam's spiritual journey, which has lasted 35 years so far and has led him around the world, began with a trip across town at the age of 14. As a teenager, James Holland played saxophone and flute. But the top 40 music of 1960 bored him. He wanted music that spoke of anguish with passion. So he went to Winston-Salem State university, one of North Carolina's predominantly black colleges on the east side of Winston-Salem, in search of somebody with whom to play music of the soul.

Four years later he enrolled at the Berklee School of Music in Boston, and there discovered the difference between an artistic adept, which he certainly could claim to be, and a true musical artist, which he decided he was not. Music, he found, was not his calling, but only a meditational fuel that propelled him into unexpected and less travelled chambers of the mind. In 1969, he joined the Navy partly to go to Vietnam to experience the war: so much of the human condition seemed to involve conflict that he wanted to find out what real war was like.

He emerged from the Navy determined to find a reality in which he could live comfortably. Despite attempts to fit into a "normal life," his path led not to the middle class suburbia where he had grown up, but to California, India, Eastern Europe and elsewhere, through an extraordinary series of what might be called living spiritual and philosophical gateways.

From masters such as Sufi master Adnan El Sirhan, Kundalini master Muktananda Paramahansa, Bhagwan Shree Rajneesh, T'ai Chi master Chu King Hung and Taoist master Ni, Hua Ching, Holland learned of a reality much more powerful than he had realized. He learned that his purpose was to become himself a living portal to enlightenment and knowledge.

After 18 months in India, San Gee Tam spent 17 years in London, engaged in intensive, high-level study of T'ai CM with master Chu, King Hung, and also teaching.

The name San Gee Tam was originally given him to by Baghwan Shree Rajneesh (Osho). In Hindi it means Celestial Music. The same name was again, bestowed on him by Taoist master NI Hua Ching, but in Chinese it means "One Whose Life Benefits All People". He is constantly inspired by and working to live up to the name.

San Gee Tam returned to Winston-Salem in early 1994. The Golden Flower school he established in Britain is flourishing there and also in Holland and Belgium. Having come full circle to Winston-Salem, now accompanied by his wife, Annukka, he is expanding Golden Flower into America, starting at what once was, and has since once more become, home.

Kumar Frantzis

Bruce Frantzis is a Taoist Lineage Master with more than 40years experience in Eastern healing systems. He is the first known Westerner to hold authentic lineages in *Qigong*, bagua, tai chi, hsing-i and Taoist meditation.

Bruce trained for over a decade in China and also has extensive experience in Zen, Tibetan Buddhism, yoga, Kundalini, energy healing therapies and Taoist Fire and Water traditions of Taoism.

Since 1961, Bruce Frantzis has followed the 3,000-year-old Taoist tradition of warrior/healer/priest by studying, practicing, teaching and writing about energy arts, including: *Qigong*; energetic healing therapies; Taoist meditation; and martial arts, including tai chi. The heart of his tradition is the cultivation of chi, the internal energy that connects the mind, body and spirit to the underlying consciousness of the universe (Tao).

Frantzis studied for a total of three years with Grandmaster Liu Hung Chieh.

In an odyssey through various martial arts that began in 1961, his ambition was always to study with a lineage grandmaster. Like other Westerners who sought this path, Frantzis was constantly thwarted throughout those years by the tightly closed door of Mainland China, a country where he was both isolated and subject to the harsh consequences of traumatic political upheavals.

His frustration was intensified by an unrelenting Oriental prejudice: the unspoken agreement that the most secret teachings should not be given to Westerners. It was not until the summer of 1981 that one of Frantzis' teachers in Hong Kong consented to give him a letter of introduction to his own master in Beijing, a man named Liu Hung Chieh (*pronounced* Lee-oh Hung Jee-eh). This letter contained potential that excited Frantzis greatly.

Until 1987, when he anchored himself permanently in the United States, Frantzis spent years alternating between Asia and the West. He earned his living by teaching *Qigong* and the internal martial arts in the United States and Europe, as well as practicing the healing art of *Qigong* tui na. In 1972, after a six-month stint of teaching tai chi in America, he departed for

India. He went first to an ashram in southern India to learn the techniques of pranayama yoga, which works directly with life energy. He practiced in the classical manner-using breath, mantras, and mudras-four sessions a day, three hours a session.

Frantzis developed a practical, comprehensive system of programs, Energy Arts Programs, enabling people of all ages and fitness levels to increase their life-force energy and attain vibrant health. Some of his Instructors have founded their own schools.

Michael Tse

HONG KONG-BORN Michael Tse has studied *Qigong* and martial arts for over 30 years with some of the world's most renowned masters. His *Qigong Sifu* (teacher), Grandmaster Yang Meijun, passed away in China in 2002 at the age of 104.

She taught him not only most of the surviving forms from the 1,800-year-old Kunlun Dayan (Wild Goose) system of *Qigong*, but also passed on the *Qigong* healing skills for which she was so famous.

With this knowledge of *Qigong*, and his study of Chinese philosophy, history and martial arts, Tse created a series of *Qigong* exercises called Healthy Living *Gong* in 1996.

Michael Tse founded the Tse *Qigong* Centre in England in 1990 along with the popular *Qi* Magazine, which gives Western readers a deeper insight and understanding of Chinese culture. He divides his time between

Hawaii, where he founded a centre in 2001, and England. He also gives seminars around the world, helping to promote the *Qigong* skills that have enriched his own life so deeply and have proven a successful way to health and happiness for so many others.

Dr Yang Jwing-Ming

Dr. Yang Jwing-Ming, is a renowned author and teacher of Chinese martial arts and *Qigong*. Born in Taiwan, he has trained and taught Taijiquan, *Qigong* and Chinese martial arts for over forty-five years. He is the author of over thirty books, and was elected by Inside Kung Fu magazine as one of the 10 people who has "made the greatest impact on martial arts in the past 100 years." Dr. Yang lives in Northern California.

Dr. Yang, Jwing-Ming instructs and demonstrates "The Eight Pieces of Brocade", one of the most popular sets of *Qigong* (chi kung) healing exercises. These gentle breathing, stretching and strengthening movements activate the *Qi* (chi) energy and blood circulation in your body, helping to stimulate your immune system, strengthen your internal organs, and give you abundant energy. With both a sitting and standing set, anyone can practice these simple and effective exercises in as little as 20 minutes a day. Known in China as the Ba Duan Jin, The Eight Pieces of Brocade has been practiced for over 1,000 years.

"I want to lead Chinese martial artists in the West back to their roots and help them regain their original high level of skill and public respect. I also wish to bring *Qigong* training to the Western world and have it accepted by the Western medical society once and for all."- *Dr. Yang Jwing-Ming*

Master Lam Kam Chuen

Master Lam is a highly accomplished practitioner of Traditional Chinese Medicine, having qualified at an early age as a herbalist and bone-setter, and establishing his own health clinic and martial arts school in Hong Kong.

It is rare to find an authentic master of an ancient art. Since the age of 12, Lam Kam Chuen has devoted himself to the internal strengthening and healing of the human body. Since those early days he has studied under masters in Hong Kong, Taiwan, and China, embracing a traditional range of studies that includes herbal medicine, the martial arts, the great religious philosophies of Chinese culture, and classical Chinese opera. He is one of the most highly trained and deeply knowledgeable experts in the art of healing and the study of internal strength currently practicing and teaching in the Western world.

In 1975, Master Lam, newly married to another martial artist, Lam Kai Sin, came to the United Kingdom. He accepted an invitation to teach Taoist Arts at the Mary Ward Centre in London, and has remained in the United Kingdom ever since. Thanks to his efforts, Tai Chi was accepted as a legitimate subject for the adult education curriculum of the Inner London Education Authority, clearing the way for the teaching of this art to thousands of Londoners and others throughout the United Kingdom.

He continues to teach, and is nurturing the art of Da Cheng Chuan with a small number of experienced students and trainee teachers across Europe. Master Lam is the founder of the first and only clinic of its type in Europe for treating people on the basis of this powerful yet profoundly natural system. The clinic, opened in 1991, can be found near the heart of London's Chinatown.

In 1994, he was invited by UK television network Channel 4 to present a ten part series *Stand Still Be Fit*, in which he introduced standing Chi Gung exercises called Zhan Zhuang. Filmed on location in China and Hong Kong, public response was unprecedented, with thousands ordering copies of the instruction booklet that accompanied the series.

Master Lam's teacher, Professor Yu YongNian, has said of Zhan Zhuan,

"My experience of the extraordinary benefits of the Zhan Zhuang style of Chi Kung exercise stretches over the past 50 years, during which time I have studied its application in hospitals and clinics throughout China. People of all ages have come to be treated for disorders that often neither Western medicine nor traditional Chinese medicine could cure: hypertension; arthritis;

some tumours, and other chronic disorders of the respiratory, cardiovascular, and nervous systems."

Chapter 6

A Basic Breathing Practice

The Abdominal Breathing Method – *extracted from Dennis Lewis 'Free your Breath Free your Life'*

If you are like most people, you are probably unaware of the extent to which the way you inhale and exhale affects your energy level. But breathing has long been considered essential to the exercises of the East. For instance, Yoga teachings include many different ways of breathing. One is "Bhastrika," known in English as "breathing of fire," whose aim is to stimulate the fundamental "Kundalini" energy. Likewise, Zen has its technique of "Su Soku Kan" (Japanese; "meditating while counting the number of breaths taken").

Several different breathing methods are used in *Qi Gong*. The ancients seem to have known intuitively that breathing conditions were related to autonomic functioning. Autonomic nervous functions are involuntary vital functions regulated by the autonomic nervous system and consist of heart functioning, digestive functioning and glandular functioning.

Our breathing changes in keeping with our emotions, such as joy, anger, or sorrow. You breathe differently when you are laughing or when you are crying. It is not possible to breathe the same way while crying, as while laughing. If you become too nervous before an exam, say, or a game, and your breathing is influenced, you are not likely to get a good result. Breathing can affect the emotional and the mental state. Many breathing methods are now promoted that seek to control feelings, mind activities, and even vital energy.

In the human body, only breathing is controlled under normal conditions, by both voluntary and involuntary nerves. This is one of the reasons why the involuntary nerves can be consciously controlled by controlling breathing. After all, breathing can become a bridge between consciousness and unconsciousness.

Improved breathing methods are effective in improving blood circulation. Proper breathing promotes the flow back through your veins and the circulation of blood through the whole body, by changing abdominal pressure. Practising breathing is an important element of *Qigong* training, but it is also important not to try too hard and not to try to do too much too soon.

Before we were born, our mother provided, through our umbilical cord, the nutrients, food, and oxygen that we needed to live. In many traditions, the area just below the navel and midway into the body is considered to be a sacred center of energy. In any event, our belly is one of the major areas that get tight and tense when we are under a lot of stress. And this greatly affects our internal organs, our breath, our energy, and our overall health. In this breathing exercise, we are going to work with "belly breathing" in order to open our belly and allow our diaphragm to move deeper down into our abdomen on inhalation and farther up to squeeze our lungs and support our heart on exhalation. This will have a powerful influence on our respiration, on the way we breathe in the many conditions in our lives.

Practice

1. Lie down comfortably on your back on your bed or on a mat or carpeted floor. Position yourself with your feet flat on the floor and your knees bent (pointing upward). Simply follow your breathing for a minute or two with your attention. See if you can sense which parts of your body your breath touches.
2. Continue to follow your breathing as you rub your hands together until they are very warm.
3. Put your hands (one on top of the other) on your belly, with the center of your lower hand touching your navel. Watch how your breathing responds.
4. You may notice that your belly wants to expand as you inhale and retract as you exhale. Let this happen, but don't try to force it.
5. If your belly seems tight, rub your hands together again until they are warm and then massage your belly, especially right around the outside edge of your belly button. Notice how your belly begins to soften and relax.
6. Now rub your hands together again until they are warm and put them on your belly again. Watch how this influences your breath. Do not try to do anything. Simply watch and enjoy as your belly

begins to come to life, expanding as you inhale and retracting as you exhale.
7. If your belly still seems overly tight and does not want to move as you breathe, press down with your hands on your belly as you exhale. Then as you inhale, gradually release the tension. Try this several times. Notice how your belly begins to open more on inhalation.
8. When you are ready to stop, be sure to sense your entire abdominal area, noting any special sensations of warmth, comfort, and energy. Spend a few minutes allowing these sensations to spread into all the cells of your belly all the way back to your spine.

This simple practice will have a highly beneficial effect on your breathing, especially if you do it on a regular basis. Remember that you can try this practice at any time of the day or night. Though it's easiest if you are lying down, you can also do it sitting, standing, and walking, and so on. It is an excellent practice to try before you get out of bed in the morning. It is also an excellent practice to work with whenever you are anxious or tense, since it will help relax you and center your energy. Over time, it will help slow down your breathing and make it more natural.

Chapter 7

What is Shibashi?

"Be kind, for everyone you meet is fighting a great battle", Saint Philo of Alexandria.

Shibashi is a Body-Mind Workout that can produce results immediately!

Most of what follows in this chapter is extracted from the words of Sifu Wing Cheung.....

Shibashi, also called Taiji *Qigong* is an easy to learn system of energy enhancing exercises that co-ordinates movement with breathing and inner focus. If practiced regularly, it will give you more energy, improve health and help prevent illness. The primary aim of practicing this *Qigong* is to gently build and regulate your vitality by enhancing your *Qi*.

This method is uncomplicated to learn so most people should be able to master the basic movements within a week or so of regular practice. Mastering the subtleties and nuances will take considerably longer, but are well within the grasp of the keen student living the modern pace of life. Within the full spectrum of possible *Qigong* methods, Taiji *Qigong* Shibashi has often been described as a relatively superficial system. However, if the nuances and subtleties are understood and practiced correctly, this *Qigong* becomes an ideal intermediate method of *Qigong* for anyone willing to do it on a daily basis. It is not one of the deeper internal methods fraught with life threatening consequences if mistakes are made; neither is it just a physical exercise. I would describe it as a realistic method for those who must practice largely unsupervised, but who wish to make real progress in the enhancement of their vitality.

If you work within any of the healing professions you will find Taiji *Qigong* an excellent adjunct to your work, because you will be giving out a lot of your energy in the form of compassion, concentration, and intent to heal, when dealing with the illness of your patients. The shibashi exercises are a particularly good way to replenish that 'giving' energy.

Tai Chi *Qigong* Shibashi is designed to improve the general health and wellbeing of the practitioner. The gentle rocking motions and stretching movements improve circulation and digestion. The chest exercises and controlled breathing are good for lung conditions and asthma. And the overall effect of the exercise is to reduce mental stress and physical tension carried in the muscles of the body. This *Qigong* is very effective and easy to learn. It is practiced around the world by over 10 million people, and is considered a national health exercise in Malaysia and Indonesia.

Shibashi is a gentle, beautiful and flowing *Qigong* exercise routine that is both a joy to do and deeply relaxing. The rhythm of 6 breaths per minute whilst practicing the Shibashi exercises, enables you to be in a relaxed and alert state. 'Shiba' means 18 and 'shi' is set.

So Shibashi means set of 18. All shibashi movement is centred on a face forward position. Diagonal side steps always return to this starting position - so in that sense it is fixed. If you can stretch your arms out to the sides and turn a full circle you have enough space to practice.

According to Traditional Chinese Medicine, we get sick for 3 reasons:

1. Deficiency of *Qi* (energy)
2. Blockages in the meridians (energy channels)
3. Yin/Yang imbalance

By practicing the first part of this *Qigong*, your level of *Qi* will increase substantially. That means your immune system will become much stronger. Your body is a great healer itself. Therefore, when your immune system is strong enough, it can heal many of your problems.

The Stress Epidemic and How Shibashi Can Help

Research has already identified the link between stress and the six leading causes of death—heart disease, cancer, lung ailments, accidents, cirrhosis of the liver, and suicide. Moreover, stress levels will likely worsen with the recent financial tsunami.

So, what is stress? In the past, when our ancestors faced danger, e.g. encountering a beast, their sympathetic nervous system would be stimulated to create a fight or flight response which resulted in dilated pupils, decreased digestion, increased heart rate, increased breathing rate, and the shunting of blood to muscles for anticipated increased activity. Nowadays, when we face stress, our bodies produce a similar response. If we are not able to balance out an overly stimulated sympathetic nervous system, our bodies will start to exhibit many chronic symptoms such as, high blood pressure, diabetes, insomnia, stomach ulcer, migraine, anxiety, emotional problems ... etc

The sympathetic and parasympathetic nervous system work together. When the activity of one is increased the other will be decreased. Therefore, one way to balance the overly stimulated sympathetic nervous system is to activate the parasympathetic nervous system.

The deep abdominal breathing, gentle tai chi movements and alpha (very calm and relaxing) mind state of Tai Chi *Qigong* Shibashi can achieve just that. Practicing Shibashi activates our parasympathetic nervous system, thus balancing the overly stimulated sympathetic nervous system. That's why *Qigong* Shibashi is so effective when dealing with chronic problems.

Shibashi Breathing

The ideal speed for breathing in each person is different. The speed should depend on your own breathing since each movement is coordinated with breathing. If your breath is shallow, you may tend to perform the whole set faster than if your breath is deep.

Beginners who have no previous training in breathing usually perform the whole set in about 10 minutes. That is about 12 breathes per minute. After you remember all the movements and their sequence, you should do it at your own pace.

When I practice this *Qigong* on my own, I usually spend about 20 minutes to perform a set. That is about 6 breaths per minute or 0.1 Hz (cycles per second). This concurs with scientific evidence that shows breathing at this pace can reduce high blood pressure.

Our body has many different rhythms. The most obvious is our heart. Its beat to beat changes produce its own rhythm. Our brainwave has its own rhythm. Our blood pressure oscillation produces its own rhythm and the pace at which we breathe produces our respiratory rhythm... etc. When all our bodily rhythms are in sync with each other, our bodies will produce a powerful resonant frequency. Studies have found that there are many positive effects both physically and emotionally when our bodies vibrate at this resonant frequency.

For human beings, the resonant frequency of our system is approximately 0.1 Hz. Studies also find that our systems naturally oscillate at its resonant frequency when we are actively feeling a sustained positive emotion such as appreciation, compassion, or love.

Most people should be able to perform the Shibashi at a pace of 6 breaths per minute (0.1Hz), after practicing daily for a couple of months. Again, doing the exercise at a comfortable pace is more important than trying to achieve 6 breaths per minute. Over-breathing may result if you are not ready and force yourself to breathe deeply to achieve this pace. Over-breathing may leave you feeling light headed.

One of the most exciting developments in Chi Gung at the end of the twentieth century and which will hopefully continue into the 21st century is the scientific testing and validation of the 'chi' component of Chi Gung.

One such test carried out in 1997 was as follows.

"The physics of External *Qi* of *Qigong* was studied using the microwave radiation component with a 3 cm wavelength spectra microwave radiation instrument. Fourteen *Qigong* masters were invited to join the experiment. External *Qi* was emitted from the Lou *Gong* point of the palm which was placed 2 cm apart from the horn antenna of the microwave radiometer. The paper describes a detection method for External *Qi* by using X-band microwave radiometry, instrument structure and experimental results"

Tests such as this one will continue to add to our understanding of Chi Gung and how it works. It will also serve to continue to make it more acceptable to the general public.

What it will do for you

Simply doing Shibashi as a gentle exercise will bring about the positive results of relaxation, gentle stretching and muscular development. It becomes more of a *Qigong* when the person practising the forms becomes aware of the life energy streaming through their arms, legs, and body. The possible results increase when the mind and breath more actively enter the process to direct and guide the *Qi*.

Nevertheless the primary purpose of Shibashi is health. The wave-like, fluid motions of the exercises stimulate the flow of blood throughout the entire body -- (Lin Hou-sheng, founder of the Shibashi movements, believes that the *Qi* resides in the blood).

In Traditional Chinese Medicine (TCM) sickness is thought to be caused by excesses or depletions or stagnation of the *Qi*. Shibashi can help to rectify such imbalances to bring about a state of well-being. Physical and emotional problems are washed away in the increased flow of the life energy of *Qi*.

Here is an example: the third movement of Shibashi No 1 is "*Painting a Rainbow.*" For this you turn the torso and arms from side to side. This regulates the *Qi* flow to all the organs of the torso (called the "Triple Burner," or "Triple Heater" in TCM). It also seems to massage and stimulate the endocrine glands—thyroid, thalamus, adrenals—and the lymph nodes in the neck, under-arms, and groin. That may help prevent the two biggest killers for all people: cancer and heart disease.

In many Shibashi forms the arm and head movements alternate from left to right, this may help to harmonize the left and right hemispheres of the brain.

Shibashi's gentle movements may be practiced by young and old alike to increase energetic vitality, rejuvenate the body mind and soul, and gain more physical agility and flexibility. It also may be an aid to lose weight, reduce emotional tension, and improve concentration; as well as gain more intuitive creative power.

Although not often mentioned in the existing literature, it may lead to deeper spiritual experiences, since in its more advanced practice, internal conscious life energy (*Qi*) may be experienced as joined to external life energy (non-local consciousness, or the divine presence in everything and everyone).

It's suitable for all groups and all ages - and you are never too old to start. My oldest pupil celebrated her 102nd birthday on the day of her Shibashi class!

Tai Chi *Qigong* Shibashi is one of the most popular *Qigong* around the world because it is effective and easy to learn. The demand for tai chi *Qigong* instructors is increasing as baby boomers start to age and as more people become aware of the benefits of *Qigong*.

Chapter 8

Fundamentals of Shibashi

"Mastering others is strength. Mastering yourself is true power." Lao Tzu

The three basic principles to always be employed in the first set of Shibashi exercises are:-

1. Full, gentle and easy breathing
2. Smooth continuous movement
3. Focus on the 'feeling' sense

Breathing
It is important to aim for very gentle and full breathing when practicing the Shibashi exercises. In the beginning, if gentle breathing is difficult, then simply breathe whichever way comes easiest.

Know that your aim is to breath at the rate of 6 breaths per minute. This is 5 seconds breathing in, and 5 seconds breathing out.

Don't hurry between the in breath and the out breath. Be natural. Breathing is an involuntary action. Wait for the 'in' breath, and then gently help it along. Wait for the 'out' breath, and then gently help it along.

Movement

The movement of the Shibashi exercises should be smooth and continuous. Do not have the feeling of

stopping and starting, even for the shortest length of time.
Keep a feeling of continuity throughout the exercises, between each exercise and during each exercise. As you move, cultivate a sense of continuousness, as if you are blending with the air around you, or as if you are like water flowing gently over rocks.

Focus

The key to success with the Shibashi exercises in positively affecting your nervous system and brain waves is by bringing your attention to your body. Try it now…..stop what you are doing and stand up. First shake each hand gently then switch all your attention to your hands. Notice what they feel like. Don't judge or assess the feeling, simply 'feel' what they are feeling like.

In this way, when you are engaging in continuous movement to practice the Shibashi exercises, simply focus your attention on your body. If this is something you are not used to doing, then begin by focusing on your hands, as you progress, expand your attention to more and more of your body until the whole body is included.

If you continue to practice employing these basic principles, you WILL begin to positively transform your state of being, your health and your wellness. Your aim should not be to learn more and more exercises. Your aim should be to embody the basic principles as you practice each one of the Shibashi movements.

Think of these basic principles as being like the foundation of a house. Once a firm foundation has been laid then the house will be well supported. You may not notice the foundations but you know they are strong when the house remains standing for generations.

Conversely you know that the foundations are not good when the house begins to collapse after a short time.

In the same way, the Shibashi exercises will be effective when you practice and include the basics at all times. This will continue to make your structure strong i.e. your posture, as you progressively develop over time.

Your posture

The Shibashi exercises will deliver benefits to you, if you stand with your feet shoulder width apart and keep an upright and relaxed posture.

However, the effects will be further enhanced, if you follow a few simple guidelines about the way you stand when performing the Shibashi exercises.

Crown of head extended

This means to imagine the crown of your head somehow connected to the ceiling or sky above you. Be aware to avoid adding tension. Just IMAGINE that your crown is connected to the ceiling or the sky.

Chin in

Very gently draw your chin towards your throat. The feeling should be that the back of the neck subtly opens up.

Drop shoulders

Over time your shoulders will drop as you consciously soften and relax your whole body. In the meantime let go of holding in your shoulders. You can also gently push them downwards, as long as you don't tighten up anywhere else in your body.

Sink the chest

Softening and relaxing, as you would do as if you are letting out a sigh, will bring the desired effect into the chest area. The chest does not need to be lifted or pushed out in any way at all.

Relax the Belly

Refer to the article on Belly Breathing in Chapter 4. Imagine the belly as the lower cavity in your trunk (the upper cavity being your chest). As you breathe, the whole belly should expand, just like a baby. There is no need to tense muscles around the abdomen.

Soften the knees

The knees are never locked. Give at the knee joints as you stand on your two feet. Allow them to bend very slightly if necessary.

Relax the toes and feet

Bring your attention to your toes throughout the day. Most people are amazed to discover that they are 'holding' or gripping on to the floor with their toes. Gripping with your toes can have the effect of tensing various key points throughout your body. Or at the very least, it will promote tensing up through the legs to the lower back.

Chapter 9

Shibashi Teachers

"To keep the body in good health is a duty... otherwise we shall not be able to keep our mind strong and clear." Buddha

Tai Chi *Qigong* Shibashi was developed by Professor Lin Hou-Sheng in 1979.

Professor Lin Hou-sheng, along with a group of Tai Chi and Chi Gung teachers, created Taiji *Qigong* 18 movements series (108 movements), combining Taiji's slow and even movements with *Qigong*s' continuous breathing and meditation. Currently, over 10 million people around the world are practicing this exercise. Today in China all students of Traditional Chinese Medicine (roughly estimated to be one hundred thousand men and women) are required by the Government to study the Shibashi of Lin Housheng. Even some Southeast Asian countries promote it as a national health exercise.

Professor Lin is a renowned *Qigong* Master, scientist and Master Healer. His remarkable credentials include Professor of the College of Chinese Medicine in Shanghai, Director of *Qigong* Research Institute in China and Honorary President of the International Society of Natural Cures.

Master Lin is well known in China and has published more than ten books. In 1980 he developed a technique for successfully using *Qigong* as the only anaesthesia needed in surgical operations: no anaesthetics, no acupuncture needles just "*Qi*" energy. His scientific studies on *Qigong* healing have been published in the prestigious journal Nature (Vol. 275,1978). Master Lin has also personally given *Qigong* healing treatments to high-ranking Chinese officials such as President Jiang Zemin.

Lin Housheng graduated from Shanghai Physical Education University in 1964. His major was in aquatic sports and Wushu (martial arts, or what is popularly called "Kung Fu"). His excellent grades enabled him to remain in Shanghai, where he took a job as a researcher at the Shanghai Physical Education Science Research Institute, which soon was closed because of the Cultural Revolution. Then he was transferred to a high school to teach physical education.

On May 6, 1966 The Great Proletarian Cultural Revolution was officially unleashed creating social chaos throughout the country. Despite the possible threat of being mercilessly beaten, forced into slave labour, imprisoned, or even brutally murdered along with his wife and infant daughter, Lin Housheng secretly practiced his *Qigong* and tai chi for many hours late into the night. This intensive hard work was to lead to many amazing achievements in the years ahead.

"In 1968, at age 29, during his practice, an abnormal feeling suddenly began running throughout his body. His nervous system suddenly became extremely stimulated. *He became excited, full of intense feelings of what it meant to be alive. The entire world around him turned into magnificent golden light. He felt his life energy (Qi), like a flowing spring, running inside his body, smoothly circulating through the Governing and Conception Vessels* [the energy meridians in the back and front of the body]. *Then suddenly, this circular flow split into two strong pathways of Qi, each flowing down from his shoulders, and out of his two palms. He realized this was exactly what his teacher had told him before about External Qi."* -- [translated from *Lin Houxing Qi Gong Shi Jie,* 1992]

On October 6th 1976, one month after the death of Mao Zedong, the insanity of the Cultural Revolution ended. Now Lin Housheng could come out of hiding and use the enormous skills that he had acquired over the years. But first he needed to answer the many sceptics in the government and elsewhere who claimed that *Qigong* was a meaningless superstitious relic from the past. To this mechanistic scientific Marxist establishment he set out to prove that *Qigong* was not some fake and fraudulent "witchcraft."

To do this he became the central subject of the experiments of a famous nuclear scientist, Gu Hansen. On March 10 1978 Lin Hous-heng projected external *Qi* from his hands which she measured with modern scientific devices. Low frequency, infrared ray modulations, and electromagnetic waves were detected. *Qi* was now scientifically shown to exist [at least the *Qi* that Lin was sending].

"*It is the first time that the physical nature of* Qi *was proven. The publication of the results of the experiment created waves within the country, aroused interest and drew the attention of numerous scientists towards* Qigong *research. Their heroic undertaking had a determining effect on the rise of* Qigong *in contemporary China."* David A. Palmer. *Qigong* Fever. Columbia University.

Sifu Wing Cheung

Sifu (Master/Teacher) Wing Cheung, Tai Chi Division Champion of the 2005 Canada Kung Fu and Wushu Championship and founder of Tai Chi, *Qigong* & Feng Shui Institute had acquired a deep interest in martial arts and had started learning northern Shaolin kung fu from his father since he was six years old. Grandmaster Cheung was a kung fu and tai chi master as well as a kick boxer, he won the Canton Province Kick Boxing Championship back in 1969.

After suffering from a serious traffic accident in 1994, *Sifu* Cheung sought the help of Master Wu Jian Hua, a famous *Qigong* healer. Master Wu was a colleague of Professor Lin Hou-Sheng at the Shanghai *Qigong* Research Institute in China. Since then *Sifu* Cheung studied acupressure, traditional Chinese medical theories and different styles of *Qigong* under Master Wu.

For the past 15 years, he has travelled to many places around the world learning tai chi, *Qigong* and other inner techniques from different teachers. He has also spent a lot of time and resources doing research on them with the latest biofeedback, neurofeedback and quantum feedback equipment.

Sifu Cheung has devoted his life spreading the wonders of *Qi* around the world. He now works as a *Qigong* healer, feng shui (the study of how *Qi*/energy flows in and around the house to bring good health and fortune to its occupants) consultant and teaches tai chi and *Qigong*. Through his workshops, he has trained hundreds of tai chi *Qigong* instructors worldwide.

"I have learned more than 30 different styles of *Qigong*. Tai Chi *Qigong* Shibashi is one of the most effective and easiest to learn. Most of my students are able to master it in just a few lessons. And many of them can feel the presence of '*Qi*' travelling in their bodies after practicing for just 3 months."

Sifu Cheung advocates entering the 'Chi Gung Mode' before you start practicing the Shibashi exercises. For beginners this generally becomes more accessible after having practiced the Shibashi exercises correctly for some time. It may also be attainable for those with some experience of meditation, or indeed to those with a naturally relaxed disposition.

Technically the Chi Gung mode is described as follows:-

Qigong mode is characterized by a brainwave frequency of 7-10 Hz. Our brainwave frequency when carrying out normal tasks during the day is above 14 Hz (beta wave). When we are relaxed and are in a peaceful stage, our brainwave is between 8-13 Hz (alpha wave).

When we are sleeping, our brainwave frequency decreases to about 4-7 Hz (theta wave). In deep sleep, it is about 0.5-3 Hz (delta wave). Since the brainwave frequency when achieving *Qigong* mode is within the lower range of the alpha wave, we should let our minds relax as much as possible before practicing Shibashi. That is why we do the Wuji stance prior to practicing Shibashi. The Wuji stance is a simple standing posture that allows you mind to return to your body. Rooting your attention in your body will draw a part of you awareness into another 'domain' completely. You will be 'out of your mind' and in your body!

Chris Jarmey

Chris Jarmey first became interested in Oriental philosophies at the age of 9, being particularly drawn to Buddhist and Daoist practices. This led him at the age of 14 into the exploration and practice of both Indian Yoga and a Chinese martial art known as Kenpo.

His interest in practices that enhance or restore health was catalyzed at the age of 11, when he suffered a serious fall from a cliff face, damaging his pelvis and thoracic spine. This caused serious pain and mobility problems by the time he was 18, at which time he applied his budding understanding and experience of Yoga and *Qigong* to successfully correct the problem.

From then onwards his interest in the healing arts developed and he embarked upon a search for those who could teach him more about oriental healing methods.

Throughout the past 30 plus years, Chris Jarmey has spent his time researching and practicing bodywork-based healing methods alongside the extensive practice of Buddhist and Daoist *Qigong*, Yoga and meditation methods.

He has been taught by several teachers, but considers himself particularly fortunate to have studied under Geshe Damcho Yonten (Tibetan Buddhism and meditation); Mother Sayama (Theravadan Vipassana meditation); Masahiro Old (Dao-Yinn, *Qigong*, Shiatsu and Zen meditation); BKS Iyengar (Hatha Yoga); Okudo Roshi (Zen meditation); Dr Norman Allen (Ashtanga Yoga) and Pauline Sasaki (Shiatsu).

Also of great value was information and insight gained at courses given by Dr. Shen Hongxun (Bu*Qi* and *Qigong*); Dr. Yang Jwing-Ming (*Qigong*); Master Mantak Chia (*Qigong*); and Dr. John Peacock (Kum Nye: Tibetan Yoga / *Qigong*). In 1975, Chris began his study of Western approaches to healing and rehabilitation, as a means to contrast and supplement his experience of Eastern methods. He qualified as a state registered Physiotherapist in 1978, with a special interest in therapeutic exercise systems.

Shortly afterwards he embarked upon extensive study and research into Osteopathic methodology. This was followed up with a training given by Carlo Depaoli in Western herbal medicine based on Traditional Chinese Medicine principles.

Concurrent with the above studies, from 1978 to 1981 he researched and evaluated the healing effects of Yoga, Shiatsu and *Qigong* within NHS hospitals and medical rehabilitation centres, with good results.

Between 1981 and 1985 Chris lived and studied in a number of Yoga centres and ashrams in India, the UK and the USA, to broaden and deepen his experience of Indian Hatha Yoga and related arts, such as the ancient and comprehensive Indian medicine system known as Yoga Chikitsa. Then, in late 1985 he founded The European Shiatsu School to offer a comprehensive practitioner training course in this effective form of bodywork. Since then, the school has become a registered charity and expanded its courses throughout the UK and the European mainland.

Chris Jarmey's adopted system of *Qigong* and Yoga has now been put to the ultimate test. He sustained a trauma that caused him to have no heartbeat and therefore zero blood pressure for over three hours. This could be viewed as a validation of his method, because he survived 'sudden cardiac death' (which normally causes death within seven minutes) by using his experience of mindful, directed *Qigong* breathing.

Chris is currently the school's Principal and Course Director, dividing his working time between giving treatments, teaching Shiatsu, holding specialist *Qigong* workshops, and writing books.

Chris was author of one of the profession's leading textbooks, "Shiatsu - The Complete Guide", published by Harper Collins. He also wrote many other books, including "The Theory and Practice of Taiji Qigong", all published by Lotus Publications and North Atlantic Books.

All of Chris' books are best sellers, having been reprinted several times in various European languages. Chris was also versed in Herbal Medicine, Nutrition and Acupuncture. He was the founder and director of the Lam Rim Shiatsu Institute based in South Wales.

Chapter 10

The Future

"In dwelling, live close to the ground. In thinking, keep to the simple. In conflict, be fair and generous. In governing, don't try to control. In work, do what you enjoy. In family life, be completely present." Lao Tzu

This book has introduced you to the powerful form of exercise called Chi Gung.

You have been shown basic practices and learnt a little about ancient masters and modern teachers.

The chapter on the history of Chi Gung has shown you that this form of exercise and movement is not a modern fashion, but something that has survived and flourished for thousands of years. To my mind if it has survived this long and is still producing results, then it must be good!

You have been introduced to the Shibashi exercises. These exercises are an easy way to manage your stress, to become relaxed, clear-headed and alert as well as generate energy.

My intention in compiling this book is to make important information available about Chi Gung and also to give easy access to a DVD about the Shibashi movements. Testimonials about the Shibashi movements are on www.mybodymindworkout.com/shibashi

I love to promote the Shibashi exercises. Whether you want to become and expert or simply start learning the Shibashi movements and enjoy the pleasure and grace they engender, the same rule applies:-
"Embody the Basics!"
Once you have embodied the basics of the Shibashi exercises, if you want, you can then work on attaining a level of expertise that allows you to refine the movements, control your breathing and maintain focus on your body, for extended periods. This can promote cells, muscle, tissue, organ systems and glands to return to normal functioning. This can potentially alleviate chronic symptoms, such as high blood pressure, diabetes, asthma, insomnia, migraine, stomach ulcer, anxiety, skin allergy, emotional problems etc.

Try the Shibashi movements and see for yourself. Purchase the DVD which has instructions, so that you can reap the benefits immediately.

To purchase the DVD go to:-

www.taichiteambuilding.co.uk/shop

To do the Shibashi movements you use your body. You use your body in a particular way.

Peter Ralston in his book '*Cheng Hsin'* – *The Principles of effortless Power*, says the following,

......"What follows are some of the most basic

observations we can make about the body and its function."

AN OBJECT

What is most basic regarding our body condition?

That it is an object. Knowing this as a fact, however, does little. Having an experience of an object, and the nature of an object, is vastly different from having a concept about it.

Rather than taking for granted that the nature of an object is known, we must take some time to consider what an object is. This opens our thinking and perceptions and provides a disposition from which new and real possibilities can arise.

Through this inquiry we also have access to experience how the fact of this object can appear as a presence, not just as something known. A great deal of this possibility resides in feeling or sensing the object that is our body, getting it now and all at once.

Increasing our awareness and sensitivity to the three-dimensional sensation of every part inside and out of our whole body brings us closer to an experience of the object. Now our attention is drawn to this object in this moment, and we are empowered to be in touch with it as a constantly changing event. It is no longer a mere abstraction or fact taken for granted. With time and practice, this presence and sensitivity can be further increased and fine-tuned.

When we experience something, we are in a very different position to it than when we simply know of it. I may know about climbing a mountain—having an image of climbing accompanied by the thought that it is hard work—but what I know by actually climbing a mountain is a completely new set of information. Having an experience of what's involved in climbing, or even just the memory of that experience, I will be much better able to design climbing gear. Otherwise, I am really just fantasizing about it, most likely using stories told to me by others.

In order to deal with this object in a more real and effective way, it appears we must first feel it, be sensitive to its presence. In our case, the body seems to function better in a relaxed state, which is actually the first or most basic condition. It is the unused condition, the body's natural state. From relaxed tissues any action can arise immediately and without preliminaries.

The principle that manifests as relaxing could be called 'letting go' or letting whatever is 'be'.

IN SPACE

The object that is our body exists in space. Just as knowing that our body is an object doesn't do much for our abilities unless we experience it and dive into its ramifications, so it is with the fact of space.

Generally we think of space as what is all around us and assume that we are observing the full extent of the matter. Most of us tend to overlook the fact that space is not just a function of the air or emptiness between objects; it is also the volume of the object. Without space, objects could not exist. We might say that space is the first or most basic ingredient of objectification. It is distance, volume, three dimensions, and objective existence.

RESTING ON THE GROUND
Standing on the ground is another thing we often take for granted. If we relax and feel the pull of the constant pressure or force of gravity that is always present on our bodies, we can surrender to it and allow it to press us to the planet.

When we feel this and accept it, we actually feel like we are standing in our feet and on the ground. But such an experience is only a thought until one has actually felt the difference. It seems that standing on the ground would be more or less the same experience for everyone, but this is not true.

There are many experiences possible within the same event. Our body structure is determined by alignment to the gravitational force, and intrinsic strength depends on channeling the compression of our tissues into the ground. Our movement depends on the ground and on our relationship to the ground, as does our balance.

IN SUMMARY
We are an object in space resting on the ground, and we are each aware of this to a greater or lesser degree. The fuller our awareness and the deeper our consciousness of this simple condition, the more ability we access in the function of our body- being. Yet it is

the nature of our mind—what we perceive and our level of sensitivity to what we perceive—that determines our actions and interactions..................

There are thousands of Qigong systems. Medical and spiritual components such as clearing the mind to reduce stress and increasing focus are built-in to all forms and styles of Qigong. Literally millions of people practice Qigong in China and around the world each day. It gives people a practical way to take more responsibility for their own health, especially for disease prevention and wellness. Qigong is not just a physical exercise system or a healing technique; it is a way of being.

Since the late 1960's many expert practitioners and teachers of Chi Gung have made the art available to the rest of the world. Recent open access to China allows almost anyone to visit, watch, and learn if they wish, the many forms of this incredible system of healing, personal growth and self-development.

Regardless of where you learn Chi Gung, the important questions to ask are, "What am I looking for?" and "what benefits do I want to gain?" Is it health and wellbeing, personal power, spiritual development and more?

My personal interest is in 'self cultivation'. This is the practice of using internal energy for personal development. Internal energy is generated by our internal organs. It is also collected from external sources, from the ground below us and the sky above us. I focus on physical practices and direct authentic communication, to enable people to access and focus their own awareness. This in turn enables them to focus on their own internal energy and the energy of others.

After 25 years of exploring and practicing self cultivation I offer the suggestion that cultivating sexual energy will affect all other areas of your life and therefore is the most time efficient method of energy cultivation to engage in.

Self Cultivation

Cultivating Sexual energy.
The following two pages are extracted from Maoshing Ni Energy Enhancement Exercises – The Eight Treasures

Around 205 C.E.[2] during the time of Master Kou Hong, who was also known as Pao Poh Tzu, there were thousands of special *chi kung* (chi *gong*) practices that expressed the different kinds of spiritual energy that people have. The importance of guiding energy is illustrated by the following story.

In ancient times, there were great floods that happened during the time of Niao (2357-2258 B.C.E.), Shun (2257-2208 B.C.E.) and Yu (2205-2197 B.C.E.). Yu's father tried to resolve the flooding by attempting to dam the flow of water. That did not work well. Yu's method was to guide the flow of water in the right direction: to the ocean.

Sometimes we use this story as a metaphor for a person who has too much sexual desire. Most people's sexual energy is too strong. Allowing it to become or remain uncontrolled, like flooding, dissipates your energy and leads to general weakness, health problems and premature aging. But just like trying to stop water, if you try to stop your sexual energy by not having sex, which is generally what religions tell you to do, this only causes the sexual energy to transform into all kinds of health problems and mental and emotional trouble. Thus it does not work well. In our metaphor, the ocean signifies Tao, the Way. So you need to guide your sexual energy and transform it correctly. Our energy comes from the ocean of Tao, and returns to Tao, the great nature.

We all know that ocean water evaporates to become clouds in the sky, which eventually turn into rain, and the rain causes saturation of lands as in irrigation or flooding. When the water is guided back to the ocean, the process of circulation is complete. The result is a beautiful, harmonized earth with productive land that provides all things for all life.

The same type of process takes place within you. Your sexual or reproductive energy is the source of your bodily energy, and it builds internally. If you just meditate every day however, without practicing physical energy conducting, your mind will become wild or scattered. You might try to control the mind with prayers or mantras, but objectively and realistically, they do not guide your energy correctly.

Standing, moving and sitting techniques are all used for guiding energy, but there are still other internal energy-conducting methods. There are many different forms of gathering and conducting energy. Because human life has different spheres of energy, it is necessary to guide and manage all of them correctly for effective and positive use.

[2] C.E. stands for Common Era and B.C.E. stands for Before Common Era. The distinction is the same as between A.D. and B.C.

Moving Forward

I trust you are finding this book useful, and if you are new to the Shibashi Chi Gung exercises, it will have opened up the possibility of starting to practice these movements. For more experienced practitioners it can deepen your understanding of Chi Gung.

The benefits of Chi Gung have been passed on by the generosity of our teachers and their teachers before them. Refinement, insights and development have come, sometimes, from over a life-time of diligent practice.

Everyone can contribute to the development of Chi Gung. Let me know what you need to further your understanding of Chi Gung and I will do my best to support your interest.

Visit www.hertstaichi.com to contact me.

Practising the simple yet profound principles of Chi Gung generates well-being, energy and vitality, our natural human birthright.

Bibliography

Yayama, Toshihiko, MD.
Qi Healing - The Way to a New Mind and Body
Kodansha International, 1993

Dr Yang Jwing-Ming,
The Essence of Tai Chi Gung - Health and Martial Arts
YMAA Publication Centre 1990

Chris Jarmey,
Taiji *Qigong* - The Theory and Practice of
Lotus Publishing revised edition 2003

Dan Millman
The Warrior Athlete – Self-Transformation Through Total Training
Stillpoint Publishing originally Clarkson N. Potter. Inc publishers 1979

B. K. Frantzis,
Opening The Energy Gates Of Your Body – Gain Lifelong Vitality
North Atlantic Books 1993

Taoist Master Ni, Hua Ching
The Complete works of Lao Tzu – Tao The Ching & Hua Hu Ching The Shrine of the Eternal Breath of Tao 6th printing 1991

Xu, Xiangcai
QiGong for Treating Common Ailments – the essential guide to self-healing
YMMA Publication Centre 2000

Paul Dong & Thomas Raffill
Empty Force – The Power of Chi For Self-Defense and Energy Healing – The Ultimate Martial Art
Element Books Ltd 1999

Peter Ralston
Cheng Hsin – The Principles of Effortless Power
North Atlantic Books 1999

Kinthissa
Turning Silk – A Diary of Chen Taiji Practice, the Quan of Change
Lunival 2009

Master Lam Kam Chuen
The Way of Energy – Mastering the Chinese Art of Internal Strength with Chi Kung Exercises
Gaia Books Limited 1991

Master Lam Kam Chuen
The Way of Power – Reaching Full Strength in Body and Mind   Gaia Books Limited 2003

Maoshing Ni
Energy Enhancement Exercises – The Eight   Treasures
Sevenstar Communications 1996

Internet

Michael Richards

http://www.mybodymindworkout.com/shibashi
http://www.hertstaichi.com
http://www.taichiteambuilding.co.uk
http://www.taichiholidays.co.uk

Sifu Wing Cheung
http:/www.taichi18.com

Professor Lin Housheng
http://www.linhousheng.com/

San Gee Tam
http://www.goldenflower.org/

Dennis Lewis
http://www.authentic-breathing.com/

Bruce Frantzis
http://www.energyarts.com/

Diabetes

1. Swing arms 8-12
2. Figure 8.
3. Side statch
4. Search for Needles.
5. Shooting arrows.
6. Water Element
7. Earth Element
8. Dantien Rub.
9. Closing Form.

Cyclical

A
1. Fire breath
2. Mind between eyebrows
3. Exhale lower abdomen sinks in
   Qi to rt side & down to Dan Tien
4. Hold, then inhale & swell lower abdomen — Qi to left side to top of head
5. Repeat 2/3 to 4.
   36 times

B
1. Inhale slowly — Qi down to Dan Tien (opposite)
2. Hold breath, direct Qi from rt side abdomen to top of head & hold
3. Exhale while abdomen sinks in — direct Qi to sink from left side to Dan Tien
4. Repeat 24 times

Printed in Great Britain
by Amazon